Essential Oils for Meditation and Yoga

1. What You Will Discover

Essential Oils for Meditation and Yoga provides information and advice enabling you to use essential oils to enjoy the experiences of meditation and yoga fully. The natural aroma of essential oils alone can reduce stress while absorbing them into your bloodstream can cleanse the body of toxins and energize the mind. Allowing you to discover a new level of mental clarity.

In this book you will also discover a wide range of powerful benefits:

1. You will discover what essential oils are how to use them for massages and aromatherapy

2. You will learn about the fundamentals of meditation, yoga, and stress management

3. You will learn how to create the perfect setting for both meditation and yoga

4. You will discover how to use essential oils to relax, unwind and create mental clarity. Helping to reduce stress levels and identify actionable solutions to your life.

5. You will discover the most potent essential oils to use and in our bonus chapter, you will receive ten blends to help you to get started.

Essential oils can enable you to create a new life for yourself using natural resources which will relieve your mind of stress and anxiety and boost your emotional state.

2. Introduction

Whether we like it or not modern society expects more from us each and every day that passes. We are constantly expected to be better at our jobs, to own every latest gadget and to be more successful than the people around us. This pressure can lead to both stress and anxiety. Stress and anxiety which can make it almost impossible for us to focus our mind and energy on finding mental clarity and happiness in our lives. Stress can also make us feel unwell and lead to serious health issues including high blood pressure and depression. Factors which having a devastating impact on the quality of our lives. However, we can find happiness, health and mental clarity by combining the natural properties found in essential oils with an effective meditation or yoga regime.

The combination of essential oils and meditation first relieves the mind from harmful stress. Stress is like a trap that many millions of people are stuck in; we can't unwind and relax because we are too stressed to discover the solutions. This book delivers that stopping point, enabling you to use essential oils to provide stress relief and take control of our anxieties.

So what are essential oil's? Essential oils are the life's blood of the plants and flowers surrounding us. When absorbed by the body these oils transfer their beneficial properties to us and deliver a range of benefits to our physical and mental health.

We can apply them to our meditation and yoga routines to create an incredibly powerful combination which not only supports us to relax more quickly but also creates a level of mental clarity. Enabling us to focus our minds on finding positive solutions to the factors in our lives which are causing us stress in the first place.

There are two key methods of using essential oils. Firstly,

you can use them as part of aromatherapy which involves burning an essential oil in a diffuser. A process which releases the aromas and molecules from the essential oils. When inhaled, the tiny nerve ends in our noise send signals to the area of brain which controls our emotions. Providing us with an instant emotional uplift and the specific physical benefits each oils provides such as treating joint ache or soothing an upset stomach.

You can also blend essential oils with a carrier oil and apply them topically to the skin using a massage which is either delivered by someone else or through a self-massage. The tiny molecules found in essential oils are small enough to enter the pores of our skin and enter the bloodstream. Once inside our bodies the natural properties of essential oils will be transferred around our bodies, delivering stress relief and the same benefits you will receive using aromatherapy. Relaxing the mind and body and allowing us to enter a calm state of deep meditation and mental clarity.

Essential oils rejuvenate the balance of the nervous system and increase our resilience to stress. They also aid the body to reach a balance and facilitate the homeostasis process. They also reverse the effects of stress and can bring our mind and body back to its balanced state. How this happens is not entirely understood but what is known is that it normalizes the body and places our emotional state and allows us to meditate and improve our emotional state.

3. What Is Yoga?

Yoga is a 5000-year-old Hindu spiritual discipline which consists of meditation, specific bodily postures, and breath control. It is practiced to improve health, relieve stress and to harmonize the body with our emotions and thoughts, helping us to feel more relaxed and boost our confidence.

In recent years, Yoga has been portrayed as a method of using the body to perform a variety of arduous and challenging body movements to lose weight and improve our health. However, this is a misconception which originates from the use of Yoga in gyms as a form of exercise to use the natural weight of our bodies to strengthen our muscles. However, Yoga is based upon the balance of mind with body. There are also various paths to using Yoga, each specializing in a detailed method which we shall discuss here:

Hatha Yoga — based upon physical postures, or asanas, the goal, is to purify the body, providing control over the internal state of our mind and preparing both the body and mind for meditation.

Karma Yoga — a form of selfless service to the people surrounding us. Using actions under the guidance of God as the Doer to relieve the mind from stress.

Mantra Yoga — relaxing the mind and body using japa, a method of focussing on the repetition of sounds to represent the inner spirit.

Bhakti Yoga — creating an unceasing worship through devotion to valuing the love and divinity everything living thing surrounding us

Jnana (Gyana) Yoga — a form of wisdom emphasizing intelligence as a method to achieve spiritual liberation

Raja Yoga — the highest path of Yoga, immortalized by Bhagavan Krishna in the Bhagavad Gita

Along with practicing yoga, you can use essentials oil to push out toxins, relieve muscle and joint ache, and improve lubrication and flexibility. Essential oils have been in use for thousands of years, many of which originate from India and used as part of Ayurvedic medical treatments. We shall discuss, later on in this book, in more detail the oils you can use to bring the body and mind closer to together.

4. What Is Meditation?

Meditation offers similar benefits to yoga but is considered to take us to a deeper level of mental clarity by transforming the mind. Using methods and techniques which are designed to develop clarity, concentration, confidence, emotionally positivity, relaxation, and the ability to identify the true nature of our surroundings. Meditation also helps us to learn the habits and patterns of our mind. Creating more positive thoughts and emotions enables us to control our attitude and concepts. Regular meditation allows us to create a focused state of mind upon a peaceful and energized status of being. Bringing us closer to nature and the peacefulness around us. Meditation has numerous physical and health benefits that include lowering the heart rate and reducing the general level of stress. Essential oils support this process by prepare us for meditation and supporting us through the process.

Meditation also helps us to connect with a sense of spirituality either towards religion or nature. Allowing us to recognize and appreciate concepts and ideas which bring us pleasure and positive mental stimulation. Experiencing these concepts and ideas helps people to 'rise above' negative emotions and events surrounding us and instead appreciate a way of life outside of their control.

To meditate effectively, the mind must go through a series of stages. These steps are widely debated with some techniques ranging from five through to nine different stages. Here is one example of a five stage meditation process:

STAGE ONE: GROSS

The first stage is considered a primer for more subtle forms of meditation. To progress through this first phase, you are required to partake in one, or several acts which are predominantly more physical. These include Physical Sensation, Chakras, Breath or Visualizations.

STAGE TWO: SUBTLE

This phase focuses on identifying and taking pleasure in natural elements. Objects of shape and form made of earth, the wind, fire, space and water.

STAGE THREE: BLISS

The third stage sees the subtle level of meditation merge into the background. Allowing the mind to enter a status of bliss, simplicity and of a single thought. The impact of our surroundings begins to lose potency as our mind and body move closer together.

STAGE FOUR: I-NESS

This stage is of individuality itself, void of personal experiences and traits. Bringing us closer to our core mind without the influence of wants, wishes or personal desires.

STAGE FIVE: OBJECTLESS

The previous four stages are referred to as samprajnata because they feature an object which is the focus of attention. However, the final phase is based on object less focus and is called asamprajnata. Creating an emotional state similar to a waking state of mind which is vast in its stillness. Allowing the body, mind and spirit to grow closer to nature in unity.

5. Creating a Soothing Environment

Giving our senses as much peace and freedom from the stresses around is essential to relax and unwind. When meditating or practicing yoga, it is vital to establish an environment that is naturally soothing not only for the body and soul but the other senses also. When creating a soothing environment for meditation, you need to find a place that you and your spirit feel comfortable. You can use your bedroom, conservatory or a location outside of the home under a tree or in an open field.

Lighting

If you are indoors, you need to create a relaxing and soothing level of lighting using as much natural light as possible. Meditating in a brightly lit room makes it difficult to relax and unwind as our sense of sight is disrupted by the strong light, making it harder for us to relax and reduce stress. The best place to meditate is outside, bringing you closer to nature and fresh air.

Noise

Finding a peaceful and quiet place is also vital to both yoga and meditation. Scheduling your time and letting other people around you know that this is your period of meditation will allow you to create an environment which is free from disruption, enabling you to find mental clarity without any distraction or disturbance. You may also want to use a recording of natural sounds such as birds tweeting or the sound of sea waves crashing together.

Smell

The aroma of essential oil burnt in a diffuser is the most powerful and effective method of helping the mind to relax and to enjoy meditation or yoga. To create a clean smell you may want to meditate as far away from the kitchen as possible. Any lingering aromas from fried onions or the smell of spicy food will make it more difficult to relax and meditate. You should also avoid meditating in a room with artificial fragrances including air fresheners. They not only feature chemicals but are entirely unnecessary. Aromatherapy provides an aroma which is full of natural compounds which uplift our emotions and reduce stress.

Clutter

A cluttered space is a cluttered mind, so it is important to try and meditate somewhere you have room to move and is safe. Being outside in a park or even on the beach are perfect places to meditate and connect with nature.

Having a soothing environment in which you can meditate or practice yoga in is essential in enabling you discover mental clarity and improve your life.

6. Benefits of Yoga and Meditation

A number of scientific studies into the benefits of meditation have begun to deliver more recognition and respect from the scientific community towards of the benefits of meditation. Examples of the findings include:

1. Increased Concentration

When we meditate or practice yoga, we are in essence exercising our brain, forcing it to concentrate on finding peace and mindfulness. Using the control of our breath and focusing our mind on a single emotion increases our level of concentration to strengthen our level of mental clarity and happiness. However, concentrating our mind on one single thought or one single part of our body is notoriously difficult to achieve and can take many hours of practice to master. This level of practice and mastery enables us to develop the skill to focus our mind more sharply and to avoid distraction. Helping us to concentrate better on our work or personal objectives. Allowing us to avoid stress by completing the things we need to maintain a quality of life which makes us happy.

2. Meditation Relieves Stress

Meditation requires the mind to enter a phase of deep relaxation. Bringing stress to the surface of our thoughts and expelling it out of our bodies as we control our breath. Relieving stress allows us to create space in our mind, allowing us to think through solutions to the problems in our lives. Practicing yoga also encourages us to stretch our muscles and release built up tension and cramp which can weigh down on our body and lead to stress.

3. Meditation Can Treat Depression

Many of us will experience some form of depression at some point in our lives. However, using meditation to relieve stress and bring tranquility into our lives is now considered a powerful method to reduce the prospect of becoming depressed. Health authorities throughout the world including in Britain are beginning to prescribe courses in meditation to help people to recover from the mental illness of depression. If you believe you are suffering from depression, it is important to seek help from your doctor. However, using meditation and yoga could be the answer many people are looking for to improve their mental health and quality of life.

4. Boosts Our Immune System

External factors can alter our immune system. For example, people who regularly do cardiovascular exercise or practice yoga tend to have stronger immune systems compared to people who tend to lead more sedentary lifestyles. It has also been recognized in recent studies that people who regularly practice meditation also have stronger immune systems. Enabling people who practice meditation and yoga to live longer and have a better quality of life.

7. Stress Management

Stress is a spiral that ratchets itself up as we move deeper into complex situations involving factors outside of our control. When we feel emotionally stressed and physically tired, we tend to produce unhealthy toxins in our bodies. Using essential oils in combination with meditation enables us to lower these toxins, relieve stress and improve our overall health. When our bodies begin to relax, we reduce the side effects of stress which include high blood pressure, aches, insomnia, headaches, and heart conditions. Essential oils also add nutrients that were part of the original plant. These nutrients cleanse our bodies, relax our mind and support our overall health.

There are other techniques which can reduce stress including the use of humor, physical exercise, hydration, power sleeping or distancing yourself from the stress. However, meditation and yoga provide a highly effective method of reducing stress and creating a level of mental clarity which enables us to both avoid stress and to use the mental clarity to find solutions and answers to the problems facing us. Allowing us to boost our level of self-confidence and create a positive outcome for any event we may face. Essential oils can be used to reduce stress and calm the mind. Allowing you to enter a calm and relaxed mental state more quickly. By being able to create mental clarity within our mind, we are also able to identify the mistakes we have made along with changes we could make to live better and happier lives. Having a clear mind is vital for us to prosper and remain healthy. You can achieve this by incorporating essential oils with meditation or yoga.

8. Depression

Depression is a biological function that affects us both on a mental level as well as a physical one. When we are in a low mood, a wide variety of compounds starts to circulate in the brain causing our brain chemistry to change. This change puts us into a depressed state where we may struggle to go outside, deal with friends, family and people in general as well as a wide range of other issues which can damage our health and level of quality of life.

If you feel you are suffering from depression or are unable to cope with issues surrounding you, it is important that you seek professional help either from your doctor, counselor or a psychiatrist. When a patient is depressed many doctors will prescribe one of many pharmaceutical drugs that will alter and replace these chemicals. However, using a range of techniques including meditation or yoga to unwind and find mental clarity may help you to find solutions to your problems and to improve your quality of life. Avoiding the triggers which cause you to feel depressed.

You can also use essential oils, essential oils impact directly on the area of our brain which controls our emotions. The natural aromas deliver an instant uplift to our thoughts and emotions, helping to remove some of clouds and darkness brought on by depression. Stress is one of the key factors which can lead to depression and is we discussed in the previous chapter, using essential oils provides a powerful opportunity to reduce stress and avoid depression.

9. Mental Clarity

When our body absorbs the nutrients and microbes found within an essential oil each and every one of them is transferred to the brain and analyzed. As this process takes place, the healing properties of the oil are absorbed by the brain allowing the cells in the brain to strengthen and grow. Improving the electrical transmission of signals from the body to the brain and then back through the body. Helping the body to increase the minds level of mental clarity. When we achieve mental clarity, we begin to development a more calm and positive mental attitude which enables us to identify solutions, enjoy nature and build better relationships with the people around us.

Creating mental clarity also frees us from stress and anxiety which pollutes our mind and clouds our judgment. The natural aromas and compounds delivered by essential oils improve each and every aspect of your life by taking control of your thoughts and increase the level of concentration and focus you can achieve. Enabling you to resolve problems and find solutions to continue you moving forwards in life. Being able to control your stress and develop the ability to find mental clarity also enables you to push yourself further, taking on new responsibilities in both your work life and personal life. Living a more fulfilled life in which, you are in full control.

10. What is Aromatherapy?

One of the best ways to enjoy essential oils is to breathe the vapors in by burning the oil in a diffuser. A diffuser will take the oils and combine them with water. Dispersing the vapors into the air as a fine mist which when inhaled will allow the essential oils to enter the body and deliver their benefits to the mind and body.

When you incorporate meditation with the healing power of essential oils, you are preparing your body for the ultimate relaxation experience. When you start to relax your body with the power of meditation you are stopping the production of negative and poisonous compounds from entering into the body. When you breathe in the essential oils, they are transferred to the brain triggering the brain to send signals to different parts of the body, affecting not only the thoughts within your mind but also the health of your body. The combination of these two processes will help increase your energy and quicken the pace for your stress relief.

11. What Is a Massage?

A massage is a process of manipulating the bodies soft tissues including the connective tissues, muscles, ligaments, tendons and joints. A massage can alleviate discomfort, relieve stress, and pain from the body. To create a massage oil using an essential oil you first need to blend the oil with a carrier oil. A carrier oil is far less concentrated than an essential oil making the massage oil weaker and safer to use. Because essential oils are incredibly potent and consist of powerful molecules applying them directly to the skin in large quantities can poison the bloodstream. Leading to nausea, vomiting, diarrhea, and other illnesses.

It is possible to deliver a self-massage which can provide a range of health benefits including helping to treat muscle wounds, joint ache and relieve stress.   If you are struggling with your meditation or yoga routine, a self-massage is a perfect way to reach mental clarity and calmness more quickly. A slow and relaxed self-massage also provides the opportunity to begin to control your breathing before you start to meditate or practice yoga. Making the process of meditation more enjoyable and rewarding.

12. Frankincense Essential Oil

The first essential to use during your meditation or yoga regime is Frankincense. This oil helps to cleanse the body of stress and anxiety, making it easier for the mind to feel calm and confident. Its aroma is woody with a spicy and fruity blend. It's origins dates back thousands of years to the Middle East as a resource to carry out religious ceremonies. However, it is now widely used in cosmetics and perfumes.

Like many oils, Frankincense can be utilized for a variety of reasons including a natural cleansing agent through to encouraging hair roots and follicles to grow. It is also considered a tonic, helping to relieve anxiety and treat an upset stomach, heal arthritis and joint pain. Burning Frankincense in a diffuser during meditation or yoga not only contributes to reducing mental stress and boost the bodies immune system, bringing the mind and body closer together in harmony with one another.

13. Myrrh Essential Oil

Myrrh oil directly stimulates the amygdalin glands, the pituitary glands and the hypothalamus. It plays a role in reducing stress and helps in focusing users minds. The scent of the Myrrh oils is also uplifting and profoundly spiritual.

The high antioxidant properties found in Myrrh are thought to be able to protect the liver from damage and improve skin health, providing a potent antioxidant to help avoid illnesses such as coughs and colds. Myrrh is used within a range of skin products to deliver nutrients and antitoxins to soothe the skin. It also features a relaxing aroma which contributes to calm the mind, allowing us to meditate and to enter the stage of deep meditation more quickly.

14. Cedarwood Essential Oil

Cedarwood is another great essential oil to support as you meditate. When you inhale Cedarwood, your blood vessels begin to relax allowing for more blood to flow through your body. Increased blood flow increases the level of oxygen which can reach the brain. Helping the mind to relax and enter a state of calmness and relaxation more easily.

Using Cedarwood twice daily will also create a natural habit of relaxing and unwinding. This repetition can become a way of life, helping you to discover mental clarity as and when you need. Enabling you to cope with stressful situations more confidently. First, in the morning to clear your mind and allow yourself to focus on the tasks of the day. Then again at night to relieve the buildup of stress you have experienced throughout the day. Allowing your body to enter in to a relaxed mental state which is ready to sleep.

15. Sandalwood Essential Oil

Using Sandalwood in your meditation ritual provides the opportunity to experience an increased level of healing throughout your entire body. It's antiseptic and non-inflammatory properties helps to ease the pain of sores, wounds and infections along with contributing to reducing swelling and inflammation in the digestive, circulatory, and excretory systems.

The carminative properties found in Sandalwood also help to relax the intestinal muscles and prevent the build of gas inside the gut. Making Sandalwood a perfect essential oil to use when you feel unwell but want to continue with your meditation or yoga regime.

16. Vetiver Essential Oil

Vetiver is incredibly powerful for helping the mind to focus and to reach mental clarity. Vetiver also provides a powerful Nervine tonic which helps to control the bodies nervous system and to maintain its health. Contributing to alleviate the emotions of fear and stress and to enter a relaxed emotional state more easily. It also provides a natural sedative to calm and relax nervous irritations, convulsions and emotional outbursts. It can also be used to treat anxiety and insomnia. Being able to sleep is essential to being to achieve a state of mental clarity. Vetiver is ideal for people with nerve problems or who find it difficult to sleep. Using it alongside meditation provides a perfect opportunity to help treat a range of medical issues and improve your quality of life.

17. Neroli Essential Oil

Originating from Ancient Egypt, Neroli Essential Oil features a range of transformational properties which alters how our mind and body works. Most notably it provides a potent antidepressant and sedative which helps to improve our morale while helping us to relax and sleep better.   It also features bactericidal and antiseptic properties which contribute to cleansing the stomach and flush out toxins from the body. It features a strong citrus fruit aroma which goes to work instantly, helping to relax and unwind quickly.

Using Neroli as part of your meditation or yoga regime enables your mind to relax swiftly and efficiently. Especially if you are short on time and want to practice yoga during your lunch break or after a long day at work. Using Neroli also provides the opportunity to increase your level of spirituality. Its powerful aroma allows many people to get back to nature and remember some of their happiest memories.

18. Rose Essential Oil

Rose essential oil features one of the warmest and most comforting aromas known to man. The aroma provides positive energy to relax the mind and to heal us mentally while bringing us closer to nature. Rose also helps to clear the mind and deliver mental clarity and calmness. Recent studies have shown that rose provides a natural reaction which relieves depression and anxiety. Boosting our emotional well-being and improving our quality of life. Rose essential oil also helps to purify the blood; its depurative properties flush out toxins from the bloodstream. Contributing to reduce the risk of suffering from ulcers, boils or skin diseases. It's nervine properties also contribute to calm the nerves and boost confidence as we come into contact with the powerful natural aroma delivered by rose oil. Allowing us to enjoy the positive experiences our meditation and yoga regimes offer.

19. Sage Essential Oil

Sage essential oil features an intense natural scent, providing emotional warmth to the body and mind. It also offers a powerful natural resource for treating digestive problems and inflammation. It also moisturizes the skin by rejuvenating dead skin cells. Sage also helps to stimulate the mind and reduce the signs of fatigue and depression, providing us with more energy and motivation to practice yoga or to meditate. Sage is also an antispasmodic oil which helps to prevent muscle spasms, helping to avoid coughs and muscle cramp. Enabling you to focus more clearly on your meditation regime.

20. Using Pure Essential Oils

As we come to the end of this book, it is important to take a step back and to spend some discussing something which many other books overlook. And that is the importance of only using pure essential oils as only pure essential oils feature the natural compounds which directly affect our brains emotions and allow us to discover a level of mental clarity. Some essential oil producers blend in synthetic ingredients, weakening the potency of the natural oil harvested from the plant to produce a larger volume of stock at a much lower price than producing 100% pure essential oil. Along with degrading their shelf life and potentially poisoning us with man-made substances synthetic oils offer far more limited benefits to the user than using pure essential oils, making synthetic oils almost worthless to use. To identify the purity of an essential oil, you should always look for the word "Pure" in the description of the oil. Such as "Pure Lavender Essential Oil". You may also see the words "Natural Grown" which also denotes that the ingredients within the oil are natural and pure.

It is also important to keep essential oils safe. Keeping them stored in air sealed brown glass bottles and out of direct sunlight is the most effective option to prevent them from turning rancid and maintaining their potency. Essential oils also have a typical shelf life of seven years, so it is important to dispose of them after the expiration date on the packaging.

21. Conclusion

Essential oils provide a powerful resource to help you relax and unwind, allowing you to create a sense of mental clarity and enjoy the full benefits of your meditation or yoga regime. Essential oils feature an intense and natural aroma which goes directly to the brain, uplifting our emotions and helping to reduce our levels of stress and anxiety. Oils can be absorbed by the body using either massage or aromatherapy. Should you want to you can combine the two using aromatherapy during a meditation routine and a massage following a yoga routine. However, when starting to use essential oils, it is important to start slowly. Taking the time to test different oils, identifying which oil best suits your personal tastes and needs. To make your experience of using essential oils more pleasurable, it is wise to use oils which feature the most relaxing and calming properties. These include sage, neroli and vetiver. It is important also to only use pure essential oils, these are oils that are free from any synthetic products and feature only natural compounds. To help you fully enjoy your time meditating or practicing yoga, it is also important to create a place where you feel completely comfortable. A soothing environment in which you can relax and unwind.

I would like to thank you for reading this book, and I am delighted that essentials oils will only help to work wonders for your meditation routine and quality of life!

22. BONUS CHAPTER: Essential Oils Blends and Fun Quiz

6 Essential Oils Blends to Help With Meditation

Blend #1

You will need:

An Essential Oil Diffuser
2 drops   Lemon
5 drops   Ylang Ylang
20 drops   Lavender Essential Oil

Blend the ingredients in a small bowl or pestle. Add five drops of the mixture to the diffuser and burn before going to sleep. The lavender will help to induce sleep, getting enough sleep is a crucial factor in being able to focus the mind and to concentrate when meditating or practicing yoga.

Blend #2

You will need:

2 oz   Spray Bottle
2 oz   Distilled Water
3 drops   Cinnamon
5 drops   Bergamot Essential Oil
1 drop   Lemon Essential Oil

Add the ingredients to the bottle and shake well. Spray 4 or 5 dashes of the formula to your pillow before going to sleep.

Blend #3

You will need:

1/2 oz	Distilled Water
3 drops	Bergamot Essential Oil
3 drops	Lemon Essential Oil

Add the ingredients to the bowl and blend. Dab the lotion onto the thigh and calf muscles and gently massage in. Perfect for removing tension from legs after a long day. Having tension in our muscles will lead to cramp and awkwardness as you try to sleep.

Blend #4

You will need:

1	Diffuser
5 Drops	Cedarwood Essential Oil
5 Drops	Frankincense Essential Oil
4 Drops	Lavender Essential Oil
2 Drops	Orange Essential Oil

Add the drops of Oil to the diffuser and burn. Releasing the mini-microbes into the air will help to create a warm and relaxing environment. The Lavender will also relieve stress and promote sleep.

Blend #5

You will need:

1 drops	Jasmine Essential Oil
2 drops	Rose Essential Oil
4 drops	Jojoba Essential Oil

Add the ingredients to a small bowl and mix well. This mixture can be transferred to a scent bottle to provide a personal fragrance. Used throughout the day it will help to keep you relaxed and calm, helping you to unwind before you begin your meditation or yoga regime.

Blend #6

You will need:

1 drop	Lavender Essential Oil
1 drop	Ylang Ylang Essential Oil
3 drops	Grapefruit Essential Oil

Blend the ingredients together in a small bowl or pestle. Add five drops of the mixture to the diffuser and burn as your meditate. The rich aromas will energize your mind and unlock energy stored in your body.

23. Fun Quiz

1. How old is Yoga thought to be?

2. Name two of the factors to creating a soothing environment

3. How many stages does meditation normally have?

4. What are the two safest methods of absorbing essential oils?

5. Name two of the two primary side effects of stress

6. Name two of the most useful oils to use during meditation or yoga

7. Which properties should look for when testing other oils?

8. On which two levels does depression affect us?

9. When we absorb the chemicals in essential oils where do they go?

10. What should you blend essential oils with?

24. Answers

1. Yoga is thought to be 5000 years old

2. Two of the following factors Lighting, Noise, Smell and Clutter are crucial to creating a soothing environment

3. Meditation is widely considered to have five stages

4. Aromatherapy and massage are considered the safest methods for absorbing essential oils

5. Two of the following factors high blood pressure, aches, insomnia, headaches, and heart conditions are considered side effects of stress.

6. Two of the following essential oils Frankincense, Myrrh, Cedarwood, Sandalwood, Vetiver, Neroli, Rose and Sage are considered the most useful to use during meditation or yoga.

7. When testing other oils, they should feature properties in relieving stress and anxiety.

8. Depression affects us on a mental and physical level.

9. When we absorb the chemicals in essential oils, they go to the brain.

10. You should blend essential oils with a carrier oil.